The Complete Vegetarian Sweet & Savory Cookbook

Delicious Sweet & Savory Vegetarian Recipes

Adam Denton

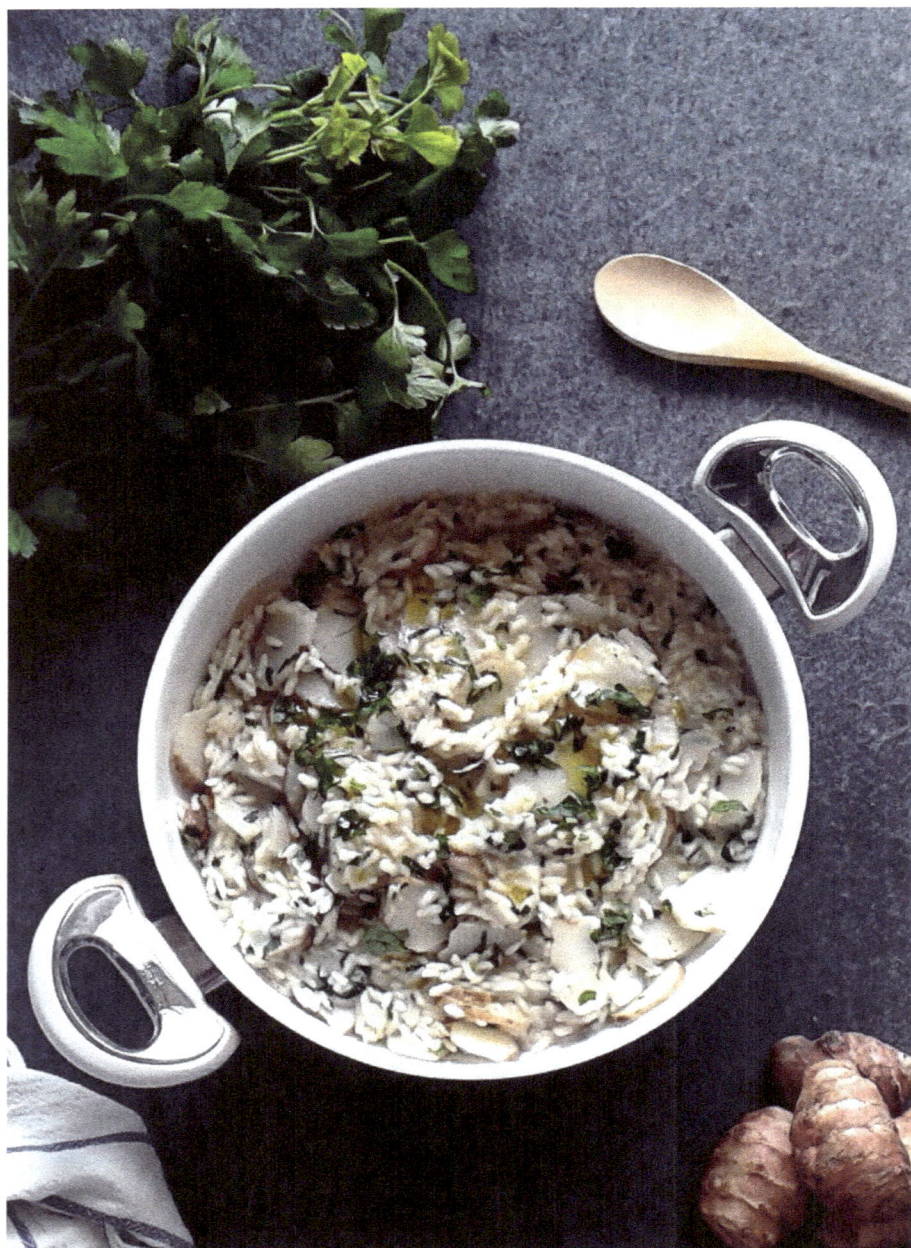

Table of contents

Lemony Easter chicks

Prep: 45 mins

Cook: 30 mins plus cooling

Easy

Makes approx 25 chicks

Ingredients

- 2 medium egg whites
- 100g golden caster sugar
- ½ tsp cornflour
- grated zest 1/2 lemon, plus 1 tsp juice
- yellow food colouring paste
- orange, black and yellow icing pen, to decorate

Directions:

1. Heat oven to 140C/120C fan/gas 1. Line a baking sheet with baking parchment and put a mediumsized plain nozzle on a piping bag.

2. In a clean bowl, whisk the egg whites until they are very stiff. Add half the sugar and continue to whisk until the mixture is becoming firm and shiny.

3. Stir the cornflour into the remaining sugar and add to the meringue, along with the lemon zest and juice, and a smidge of yellow food colouring paste. Whisk again until you have a very thick, firm and glossy pale yellow meringue.

4. Carefully spoon the meringue into the piping bag. Push any air out of the top and tightly twist the opening to seal. Pipe about 25 thumb-sized dollops onto your baking sheet – if possible, try to make them wider at the base than the top, resembling a chick's body and head. Leave a gap between each chick to allow for expanding when cooking.

5. Cook in the oven for 30 mins until they are crisp, firm and come off the baking parchment easily. Leave to cool on a wire rack.

6. To decorate, use the orange icing pen to make a V-shaped beak, and a black icing pen for eyes and feet. The yellow icing pen can be used to decorate fluffy hair on the chick's head and/or wings. Will keep for up to 1 week in an airtight container.

Mini chocolate cheesecakes

Prep: 20 mins

Cook: 30 mins

Easy

Makes 12

Ingredients

- 14 milk chocolate digestive biscuits, finely crushed
- 100g butter, melted

For the filling

- 500g tub ricotta
- 3 eggs, beaten
- 1 tsp vanilla extract
- 200g cheap dark chocolate, broken into chunks and melted
- 125g icing sugar
- 36 mini chocolate eggs

Directions:

1. Heat oven to 150C/130C fan/gas 2. Line the holes of a muffin tin with 12 paper muffin cases. Put the biscuits in a food bag and bash to small crumbs with the end of a rolling pin. Tip into a bowl, stir in the melted butter until the crumbs are nicely coated, then spoon between the paper cases. Press down into the bottoms to make a firm base.

2. To make the filling, put the ricotta, eggs, vanilla and melted chocolate in a large mixing bowl. Sift in the icing sugar. Beat everything together with an electric whisk or a wooden spoon until very well combined. Spoon into the paper cases right up to the tops, then tap the whole tin on the bench to get rid of any air bubbles. Bake for 30 mins, then remove from the oven and gently push 3 mini eggs into the top of each cheesecake. Let the cheesecakes cool completely before serving. Can be kept in the fridge for up to 3 days.

Christmas pudding cake pops

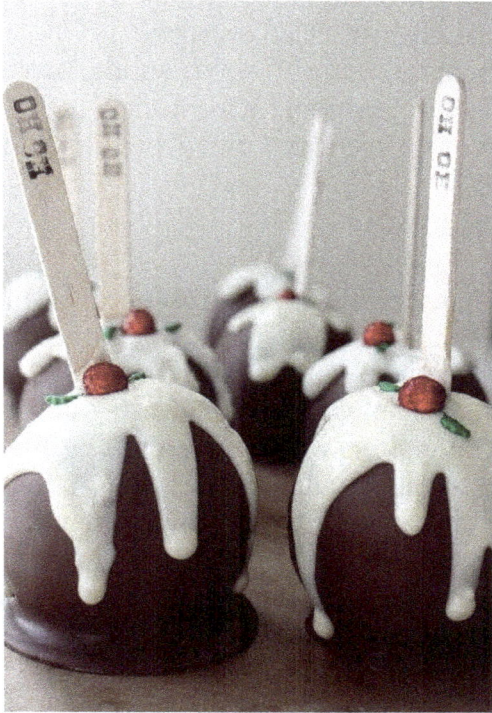

Prep: 1 hr and 30 mins - 1 hr and 50 mins

Cook: 20 mins

More effort

Makes 10 cake pops

Ingredients

- 200g madeira cake
- 140g-160g white chocolate (see Tip)
- 1 orange, zest finely grated To decorate
- 300g dark chocolate, 60-70% cocoa solids, broken into chunks
- 50g white chocolate, broken into chunks
- sugar holly decorations or red and green writing icing

Directions:

1. Pulse the madeira cake in a food processor until you have fine crumbs. Melt the white chocolate in a bowl over just simmering water or in the microwave. Shop bought madeira cake can vary in texture so you may need to add a little extra melted white chocolate to make the mixture stick into balls. Stir the orange zest into the chocolate, then work the chocolate into the crumbs using your hands.

2. Form into 10 small truffle-sized balls, then roll gently in your palms to smooth the surface. Arrange the balls on a baking parchment-lined dinner plate. Refrigerate for 30 minutes to allow the mixture to set.

3. Melt the dark chocolate in a microwave or over a bowl of just simmering water. Dip a lolly stick into the melted chocolate about 1.5cm in and poke half way into a cake ball. Repeat with the remaining balls. Put them back on the plate. Return to the fridge for five minutes.

4. Dip the cake pops one at a time into the melted chocolate, allowing any excess chocolate to drip off and spin the pops to even out the surface. Poke the pops into a piece of polystyrene or cake pop holder if you have one, keeping the pops apart. Allow to set for about half an hour.

5. Heat the white chocolate in a microwave or over a pan of simmering water. Allow to cool for a few minutes until it has a thick, runny consistency. If the chocolate is too hot,

it will melt the dark chocolate underneath so make sure you do not overheat it. Spoon a small amount on top of the cake pops and tip them back and forth so that it runs down the sides a little. If you have holly decorations, set one on each pop. If using writing icing, wait for another 20 minutes or so until the white chocolate has set. To avoid a bloom on the chocolate, cover the cake pops in chocolate on the day you want to eat them– or the day before at the earliest.

6. Pipe on holly leaves with the green icing and two little dots for berries using the red. Once finished, store them in a cool place, though not the fridge

Creamy veggie risotto

Prep:10 mins

Cook:30 mins

Easy

Serves 2 adults and 2-3 children

Ingredients

- 1 tbsp olive oil
- 1 onion, chopped
- 1 parsnip, finely diced
- 2 medium carrots, finely diced
- 350g risotto rice, such as arborio
- 1 bay leaf
- 1.2l hot vegetable or chicken stock
- 140g frozen pea or petit pois
- 50g parmesan (or vegetarian alternative), grated

Directions:

1. Heat the oil in a large shallow pan. Tip in the onion, parsnip and carrots, cover and gently fry for 8 mins until the onion is very soft.

2. Stir in the rice and bay leaf, then gently fry for another 2-3 mins until the rice starts to turn seethrough around the edges. Add 300ml of the stock and simmer over a gentle

heat, stirring until it has all been absorbed. Carry on adding the hot stock, a ladleful at a time, letting it be absorbed before adding more. Continue until the rice is just cooked and all the stock has been used, adding a little more water or stock if needed. This will take 18-20 mins.

3. Remove the bay leaf from the cooked risotto and stir in the peas. Heat through for a few mins, then add most of the Parmesan and season to taste. Sprinkle with the remaining Parmesan and serve.

Pumpkin risotto

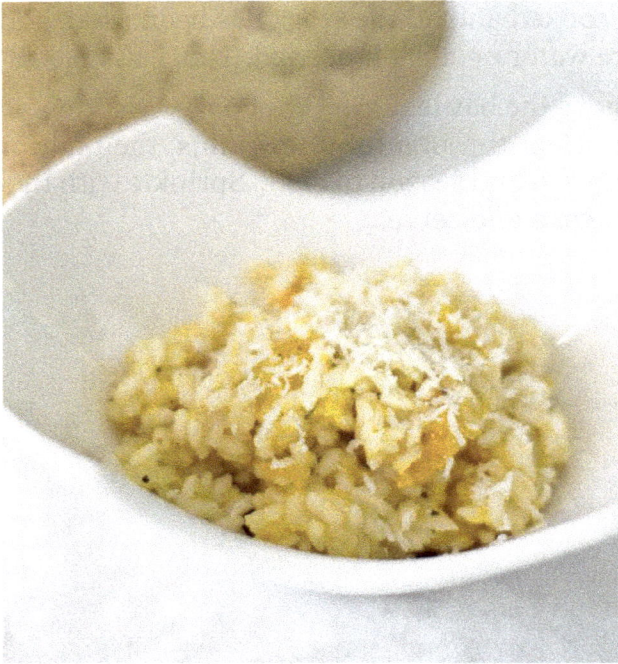

Prep:30 mins

Cook:1 hr

Easy

Serves 4

Ingredients

• 1 small pumpkin or butternut squash- after peeling and scraping out the seeds, you need about 400g/14oz
• 1 tbsp olive oil, plus a drizzle for the pumpkin
• 2 garlic cloves
• 8 spring onions
• 25g butter
• 200g risotto rice
• 2 tsp ground cumin
• 1l hot vegetable stock, plus extra splash if needed
• 50g grated parmesan (or vegetarian alternative)
• small handful coriander, roughly chopped

Directions:

1. Heat oven to 180C/160C fan/ gas 4. Chop up the pumpkin or squash into 1.5cm cubes (kids- ask for help if it's slippery). Put it on a baking tray, drizzle over some oil, then roast for 30 mins.

2. While the pumpkin is roasting, you can make the risotto. Put the garlic in a sandwich bag, then bash lightly with a rolling pin until it's crushed.

3. Cut up the spring onions with your scissors.

4. Heat 1 tbsp oil with the butter in your pan over a medium heat – not too hot. Add the spring onions and garlic. Once the onions are soft but not getting brown, add the rice and cumin. Stir well to coat in the buttery mix for about 1 min.

5. Now add half a cup of the stock, and stir every now and then until it has all disappeared into the rice. Carry on adding and stirring in a large splash of stock at a time, until you have used up all the stock– this will take about 20 mins.

6. Check the rice is cooked. If it isn't, add a splash more stock, and carry on cooking for a bit. Once the rice is soft enough to eat, gently stir in the grated cheese, chopped coriander and roasted pumpkin.

Vietnamese veggie hotpot

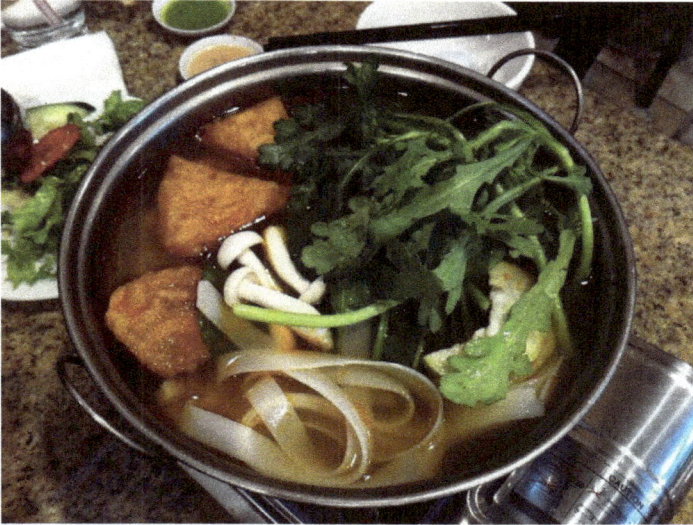

Prep: 5 mins

Cook: 20 mins

Easy

Serves 4

Ingredients
- 2 tsp vegetable oil
- thumb-size piece fresh root ginger, shredded

- 2 garlic cloves, chopped
- ½ large butternut squash, peeled and cut into chunks
- 2 tsp soy sauce
- 2 tsp soft brown sugar
- 200ml vegetable stock
- 100g green bean, trimmed and sliced
- 4 spring onions, sliced
- coriander leaves and cooked basmati or jasmine rice, to serve

Directions:

Heat the oil in a medium-size, lidded saucepan. Add the ginger and garlic, then stir-fry for about 5 mins. Add the squash, soy sauce, sugar and stock. Cover, then simmer for 10 mins. Remove the lid, add the green beans, then cook for 3 mins more until the squash and beans are tender. Stir the spring onions through at the last minute, then sprinkle with coriander and serve with rice.

Baileys banana trifles

Prep: 10 mins

Easy

Serves 6

Ingredients

• 300g pot extra-thick double cream
• 7 tbsp Baileys
• 6 chocolate brownies (about 250g/9oz), broken up, or use crumbled chocolate biscuits or loaf cake
• 3 bananas, sliced
• 500g pot vanilla custard
• 6 tbsp toffee sauce
• 25g chocolate, grated

Directions:

Mix the cream with 1 tbsp Baileys, and set aside. Divide the brownie pieces between 6 glasses, then drizzle each with 1 tbsp Baileys. Top with the sliced bananas, custard and Baileys cream, dividing equally, then drizzle with toffee sauce and finish with grated chocolate. Can be made a few hours ahead.

Christmas biscuits

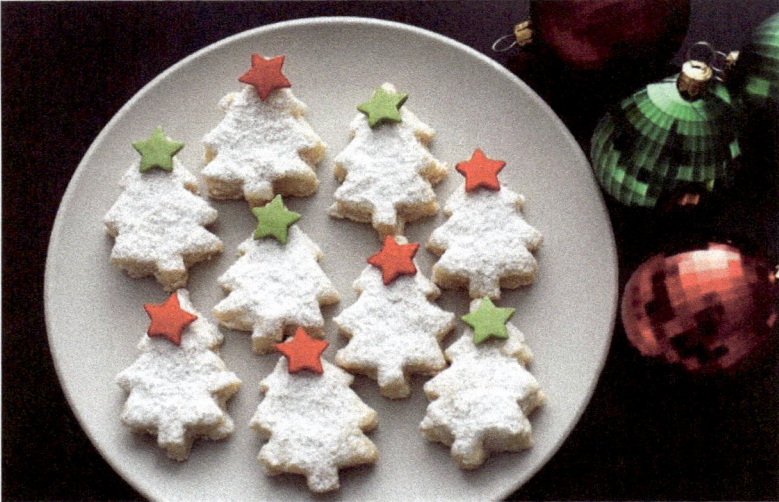

Prep:40 mins

Cook:15 mins Plus chilling

Easy

Makes 30-40 depending on size

Ingredients
• 175g dark muscovado sugar
• 85g golden syrup
• 100g butter

- 3 tsp ground ginger
- 1 tsp ground cinnamon
- 350g plain flour, plus extra for dusting
- 1 tsp bicarbonate of soda
- 1 egg, lightly beaten To finish
- 100g white chocolate
- edible silver balls

Directions:

1. Heat the sugar, golden syrup and butter until melted. Mix the spices and flour in a large bowl. Dissolve the bicarbonate of soda in 1 tsp cold water. Make a well in the centre of the dry Ingredients, add the melted sugar mix, egg and bicarbonate of soda. Mix well. At this stage the mix will be soft but will firm up on cooling.

2. Cover the surface of the biscuit mix with wrapping and leave to cool, then put in the fridge for at least 1 hr to become firm enough to roll out.

3. Heat oven to 190C/170C fan/gas 5. Turn the dough out onto a lightly floured surface and knead briefly. (At this stage the dough can be put into a food bag and kept in the fridge for up to a week.) Cut the dough in half. Thinly roll out one half on a lightly floured surface. Cut into shapes with cutters, such as gifts, trees and hearts, then transfer to baking sheets, leaving a little room for them to spread. If you plan to hang the biscuits up, make a small hole in the top of each one using a skewer. Repeat with remaining dough.

4. Bake for 12-15 mins until they darken slightly. If the holes you have made have closed up, remake them while the biscuits are warm and soft using a skewer.

Cool for a few mins on the baking sheets, then transfer to a wire rack to cool and harden up completely.

5. Break up the chocolate and melt in the microwave on Medium for 1-2 mins, or in a small heatproof bowl over simmering water. Drizzle the chocolate over the biscuits, or pipe on shapes or names, then stick a few silver balls into the chocolate. If hung up on the tree, the biscuits will be edible for about a week, but will last a lot longer as decorations.

Cheese roll-ups

Prep:30 mins

Cook:25 mins

Easy

Makes 6

Ingredients
- 200g self-raising flour, plus extra for dusting
- 50g butter, softened
- 1 tsp paprika
- 100-125ml/3½-4fl oz milk
- 50g ready-grated mature cheddar

Directions:
1. Heat oven to 220C/200C fan/gas 7. Put the flour and butter in a bowl and rub them together with your fingers. Rubbing in mixture with cold butter is hard and tiring on young fingers, so use slightly softened butter – but not so soft that it is oily. Now stir in the paprika and mix again.

2. Add 100ml milk and mix with a fork until you get a soft dough. Add a splash more milk if the dough is dry. This process will teach you how to feel the dough and

decide if it needs more liquid. You can always add more milk if required.

3. On a lightly floured surface, roll out the dough like pastry to about 0.5cm thick. Try to keep a rectangular shape. Only roll in one direction, and roll and turn, roll and turn – by keeping the dough moving, you avoid finding it stuck at the end.

4. Sprinkle the grated cheese on top, then roll up like a sausage along the long side. Cut into 12 thick rings using a table knife. Get an adult to show you how to hold the dough with one hand and cut straight through with the other.

5. Line the baking tray with baking parchment. Place the roll-ups on the parchment, cut-side down, almost touching each other, making sure that you can see the spiral. Get an adult to put them in the oven for you and bake for 20-25 mins until golden and melty. Ask an adult to remove them from the oven, then leave to cool. The cheese roll-ups will keep for up to 3 days in an airtight container.

Fright Night fancies

Prep:25 mins

No cook

Easy

Serves 12

Ingredients

• 12 ready-made vanilla cupcakes or fairy cakes, or make your own (see tip)
• 2 x 410g cans apricot halves in light syrup, drained (reserve the syrup)
• 100g raspberry jam
• a little icing sugar or cornflour, for dusting
• 500g pack ready-to-roll white fondant icing
• black icing pen

Directions:

1. Remove the cakes from their paper cases – if the tops are rounded, trim them with a serrated knife to make a flat surface. Flip the cakes over and arrange on a large board or cake stand. Brush the cakes all over with the syrup from the drained apricots, then place 1 tsp

jam on top of each cake. Put an apricot half on top of the jam, rounded- side facing up.

2. Clean your work surface, then dust with a little icing sugar or cornflour. Roll out the icing to the thickness of a 50p piece – it will be easier if you work with half at a time, keeping the remaining icing well wrapped so it doesn't dry out. Use a 12cm fluted cookie cutter to stamp out 12 circles and, as soon as you cut each one, drape it over a cake. Draw on spooky faces using the black icing pen, then serve. Can be made up to a day ahead; eat leftover cakes within 1 day.

Courgette muffins

Prep:35 mins

Cook:25 mins Plus cooling

Easy

Makes 12

Ingredients
• 50g courgette, cut into chunks
• 1 apple, peeled and quartered
• 1 orange, halved
• 1 egg
• 75g butter, melted
• 300g self-raising flour
• ½ tsp baking powder
• ½ tsp cinnamon
• 100g golden caster sugar
• handful of sultanas
• 1 tub soft cheese mixed with 3 tbsp icing sugar, to make icing

Directions:
1. Brush the muffin tin with oil. Ask your grown-up helper to switch the oven to 190C/ 170C fan/gas 5.

2. Grate the courgettes and put them in a large bowl. Grate the apple and add to the bowl. Squeeze the orange and add the juice to the bowl.

3. Break the egg into a bowl; if any bits of shell get in, scoop them out with a spoon. Stir the butter and egg into the courgette and apple mix.

4. Sieve the flour, baking powder and cinnamon into the bowl. Add the sugar and sultanas.

5. Mix with a spoon until everything is combined, but don't worry if it is lumpy.

6. Spoon the mixture into the tin. Ask your helper to put it in the oven and cook for 20-25 mins. Cool in the tin, then spread some icing on each.

Borlotti Bean Soup

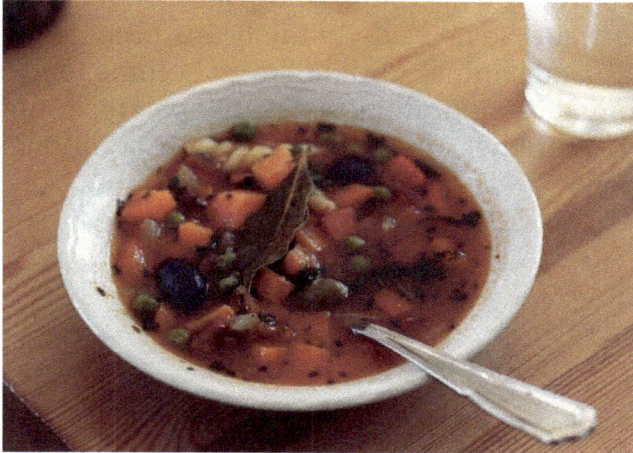

Ingredients

1 pound borlotti beans, sorted and rinsed

2 quarts veggie stock

1 medium red onion, diced

5 cloves of garlic, peeled and smashed

2 tsp. sea salt

1/4 tsp white pepper

2 medium sweet potatoes, diced

1 pound frozen, sliced parsnips

3/4 cup chopped sun-dried tomatoes*

1-2 tsp dried dill

3-4 tbsp fresh, minced parsley

Directions:

Place the beans, stock, onion, garlic, sea salt and pepper in a pot Cook them over low-medium heat. Simmer for 3-4 hours, or longer, add water as needed. As the beans become soft, add the sweet potato and simmer until potatoes become tender. Add the carrots, tomatoes and dill. Cook the parsnips until heated thoroughly. Add the parsley, season with additional salt and white pepper.

Lentil Soup

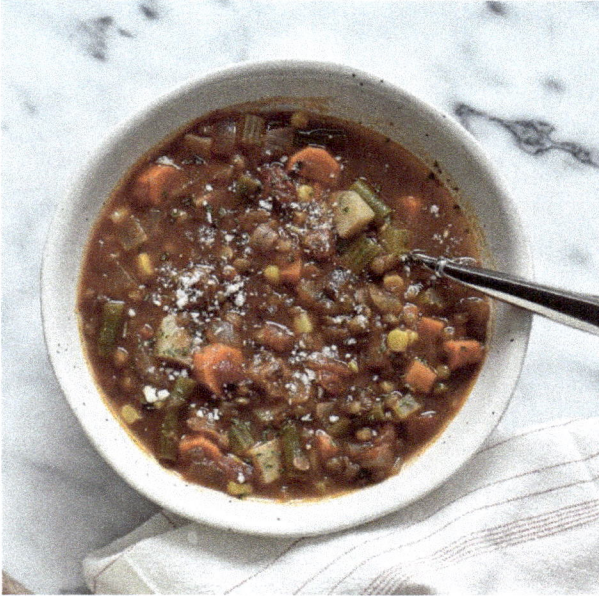

Ingredients

1/2 pound lentils, sorted and rinsed

½ pound fava beans, sorted and rinsed

2 quarts veggie broth

1 medium red onion, diced

6 cloves of garlic, peeled and smashed

tsp. sea salt

1/4 tsp white pepper

2 medium potatoes, diced

1 pound frozen, sliced carrots

3/4 cup chopped sun-dried tomatoes*

1-2 tsp dried dill

3-4 tbsp fresh, minced parsley

Directions:

Place the beans, broth, red onion, garlic, sea salt and pepper in a pot Cook them over low-medium heat. Simmer for 3-4 hours, or longer, add water as needed. As the beans become soft, add the potato and simmer until potatoes become tender. Add the carrots, tomatoes and dill. Cook the carrots until heated thoroughly. Add the parsley, season with additional salt and white pepper.

Triple Bean Soup

Ingredients

1/2 pound borlotti beans, sorted and rinsed

¼ pound great northern beans, sorted and rinsed

¼ pound kidney beans, sorted and rinsed

2 quarts veggie broth

1 medium onion, diced

5 cloves of garlic, peeled and smashed

2 tsp. sea salt

1/4 tsp rainbow peppercorns

2 medium potatoes, diced

1 pound frozen, sliced carrots

3/4 cup chopped sun-dried tomatoes*

1-2 tsp dried dill

3-4 tbsp fresh, minced parsley

Directions:

Place the beans, stock, onion, garlic, sea salt and pepper in a pot Cook them over low-medium heat. Simmer for 3-4 hours, or longer, add water as needed. As the beans become soft, add the potato and simmer until potatoes become tender. Add the carrots, tomatoes and dill. Cook the carrots until heated thoroughly. Add the parsley, season with additional salt and peppercorns.

Parsnips and Summer Squash Soup

Ingredients

1 medium summer squash (1 lb of peeled and cubed butternut squash)

1/2 medium red onion, diced

½ medium yellow onion, diced

2/3 lb parsnips, peeled and cut into chunks

1 carrot, peeled and sliced

3 cups vegetable broth

1 bay leaf

1 tsp sea salt

1 tsp white pepper

1/4 tsp dried ground sage

½ can almond milk

Directions:

Combine the squash, red and yellow onion, parsnips, apple, broth and bay leaf in a slow cooker. Cover and cook on low for about 6 hours or until veggies are soft. Take out the bay leaf and discard. Transfer these ingredients to a blender and blend until smooth Pour it back to the slow cooker Season with salt, pepper & sage Pour the almond milk. Add more salt and pepper to taste.

Butternut Squash and Apple Soup

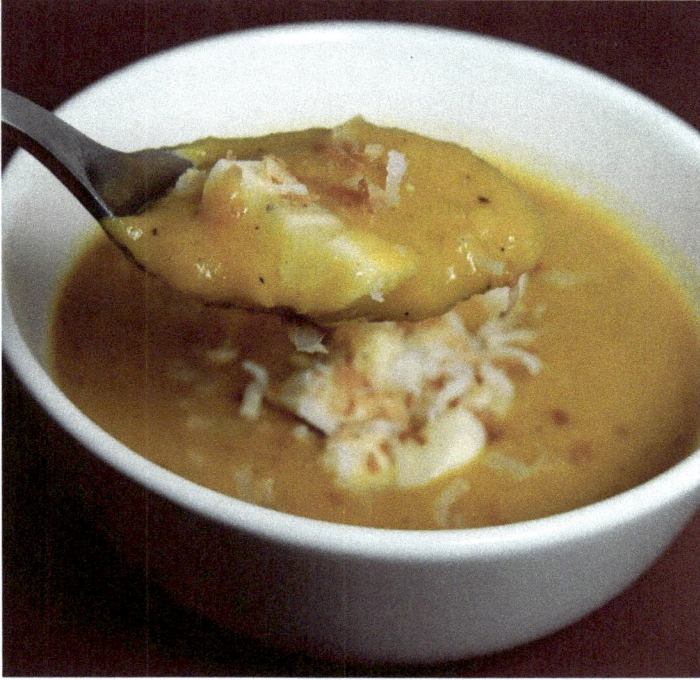

Ingredients

1 medium butternut squash (1 lb of peeled and cubed butternut squash)

1 medium red onion, diced

2/3 lb parsnips, peeled and cut into chunks

1 Washington apple, peeled and sliced

3 cups vegetable stock

1 bay leaf

1 tsp sea salt

1 tsp white pepper

1/4 tsp dried ground sage

½ can coconut milk

Directions:

Combine the squash, red onion, carrots, apple, stock and bay leaf in a slow cooker. Cover and cook on low for about 6 hours or until veggies are soft. Take out the bay leaf and discard. Transfer these ingredients to a blender and blend until smooth Pour it back to the slow cooker Season with sea salt, pepper & sage Pour the coconut milk.

Summer Squash and Apple Soup

Ingredients

1 medium summer squash (1 lb of peeled and cubed butternut squash)

1 medium red onion, diced

2/3 lb carrots, peeled and cut into chunks

1 Fuji apple, peeled and sliced

3 cups vegetable broth

1 tsp. red curry powder

1 tsp sea salt

1 tsp black pepper

1/4 tsp cumin

½ can coconut milk

Directions:

Combine the squash, onion, carrots, apple, broth and curry powder in a slow cooker. Cover and cook on low for about 6 hours or until veggies are soft. Transfer these ingredients to a blender and blend until smooth Pour it back to the slow cooker Season with salt, pepper & cumin Pour the coconut milk. Add more salt and pepper to taste.

Chinese Butternut Squash Soup

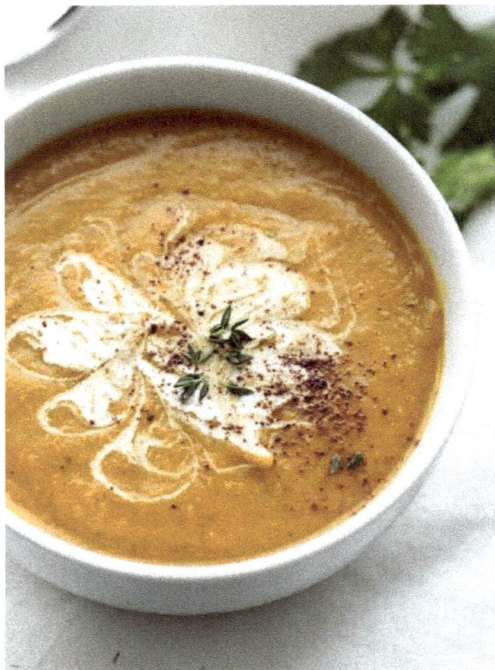

Ingredients

1 medium butternut squash (1 lb of peeled and cubed butternut squash)

1 medium red onion, diced

2/3 lb carrots, peeled and cut into chunks

1 pears, peeled and sliced

3 cups vegetable broth

2 tbsp. sesame seed oil

1 tsp sea salt

1 tsp Sichuan peppercorns

1/4 tsp dried ground sage

½ can almond milk

Directions:

Combine the squash, onion, carrots, pear & broth in a slow cooker. Cover and cook on low for about 6 hours or until veggies are soft. Take out the bay leaf and discard. Transfer these ingredients to a blender and blend until smooth Pour it back to the slow cooker Season with salt, pepper, sesame oil & Sichuan peppercorns Pour the almond milk. Add more salt and pepper to taste.

Pinto Beans and Olives Tortilla Soup

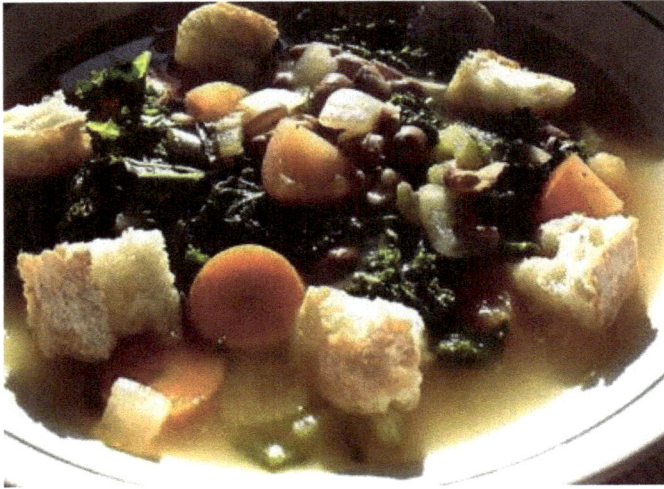

Ingredients:

1 teaspoon extra-virgin olive oil

1/2 cup chopped red onions

6 cloves garlic, minced

1 cup vegetable broth

1 cup vegetable stock

1 cup salsa

1 14-ounce can pinto beans

5 pcs. black olives

5 pcs. capers

1 green bell pepper, chopped

1/2 teaspoon salt

1 avocado, chopped

1/2 cup loosely-packed cilantro

Optional:

1/2 cup crumbled corn tortilla chips

Add olive oil to a pan and heat it to medium.

Directions:

Add onions and garlic to saucepan and sauté until softened. Add the stock, salsa, bell peppers, capers, olives beans, and salt. Bring to a boil over high heat. Reduce to low and simmer for 5 minutes. Garnish with half of the avocado, cilantro, and tortilla chips.

Butterbean Taco Soup

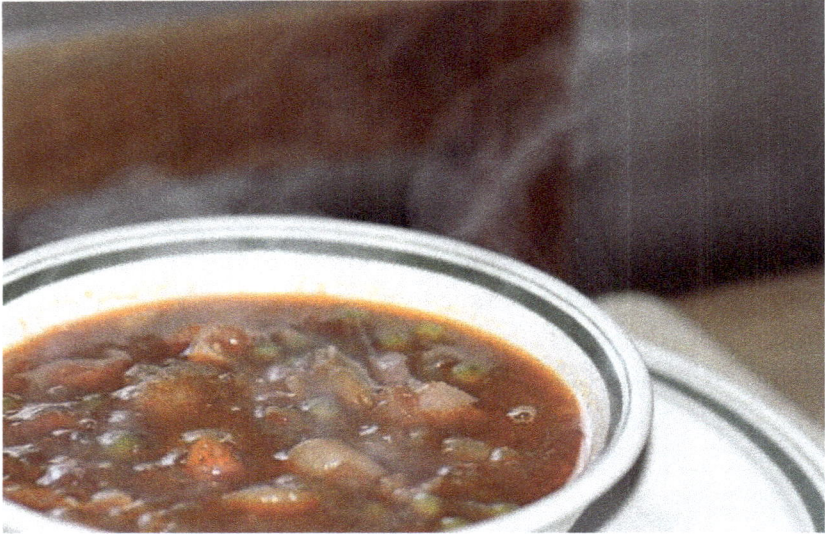

Ingredients:

1 teaspoon extra-virgin olive oil

1/2 cup chopped red onions

8 cloves garlic, minced

1 lime, peeled

1 cup vegetable broth

1 cup vegetable stock

1 cup salsa

1 14-ounce can butterbeans

1 green bell pepper, chopped

1/2 teaspoon salt

1 avocado, chopped

1/2 cup loosely-packed cilantro

Directions:

Add red onions and garlic to saucepan and sauté until softened. Add the stock, salsa, bell peppers, beans, lime, and salt. Bring to a boil over high heat. Reduce to low and simmer for 5 minutes. Garnish with half of the avocado, cilantro, and tortilla chips. Remove the lime

Jalapeno and Soybean Taco Soup

Ingredients:

1 teaspoon olive oil

1/2 cup chopped red onions

10 cloves garlic, minced

1 cup vegetable broth

1 cup vegetable stock

1 cup salsa

1 14-ounce can soy beans

1 green bell pepper, chopped

1 Anaheim pepper, coarsely chopped

2 jalapeno peppers, coarsely chipped

1/2 teaspoon salt

1 avocado, chopped

1/2 cup loosely-packed cilantro

Directions:

Optional: 1/2 cup crumbled corn tortilla chips Add olive oil to a pan and heat it to medium. Add red onions and garlic to saucepan and sauté until softened. Add the stock, salsa, bell peppers, Anaheim peppers, jalapeno, beans, and salt. Bring to a boil over high heat. Reduce to low and simmer for 5 minutes. Garnish with half of the avocado, cilantro, and tortilla chips.

Sweet Potato and Apple Latkes

Preparation time: 5 minutes

Cooking time: 15 minutes

Servings: 4

Ingredients:

1 large sweet potato, peeled, grated

1/2 of medium white onion, diced

1 apple, peeled, cored, grated

2 tablespoons spelt flour

1 tablespoon arrowroot powder

½ teaspoon cracked black pepper

1 teaspoon salt

1 teaspoon turmeric

1 tablespoon olive oil and more for frying

Tahini lemon drizzle, for serving

Directions:

Wrap grated potato and apple in a cheesecloth, then squeeze moisture as much as possible and then place in a bowl. Add remaining ingredients and then stir until combined. Take a skillet pan, place it over medium-high heat, add oil and when hot, drop in prepared batter, shape them into a round patty and cook for 4 minutes per side until crispy and brown. Serve latkes with Tahini lemon drizzle.

Vegan Breakfast Sandwich

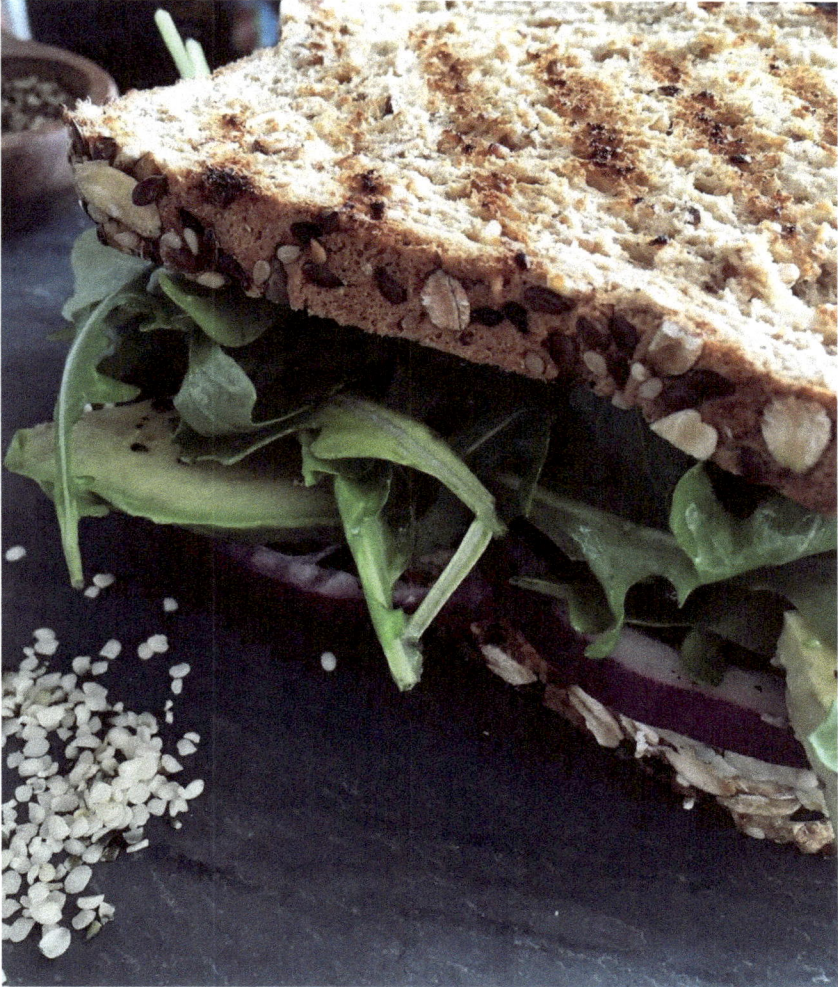

Preparation time: 15 minutes

Cooking time: 8 minutes

Servings: 3

Ingredients:

1 cup of spinach

6 slices of pickle

14 oz tofu, extra-firm, pressed

2 medium tomatoes, sliced

1/2 teaspoon garlic powder

¼ teaspoon ground black pepper

1/2 teaspoon black salt

1 teaspoon turmeric

1 tablespoon coconut oil

2 tablespoons vegan mayo

3 slices of vegan cheese

6 slices of gluten-free bread, toasted

Directions:

Cut tofu into six slices, and then season its one side with garlic, black pepper, salt, and turmeric. Take a skillet pan, place it over medium heat, add oil and when hot, add seasoned tofu slices in it, season side down, and cook for 3 minutes until crispy and light brown. Then flip the tofu slices and continue cooking for 3 minutes until browned and crispy. When done, transfer tofu slices on a baking sheet, in the form of a set of two slices side by side, then top each set with a cheese slice and broil for 3 minutes until cheese has melted. Spread mayonnaise on both sides of slices, top with two slices of tofu, cheese on the side, top with spinach, tomatoes, pickles, and then close the sandwich. Cut the sandwich into half and then serve.

Tofu Scramble

Preparation time: 5 minutes

Cooking time: 18 minutes

Servings: 4

Ingredients:

For The Spice Mix:

1 teaspoon black salt

1/4 teaspoon garlic powder

1 teaspoon red chili powder

1 teaspoon ground cumin

3/4 teaspoons turmeric

2 tablespoons nutritional yeast

For The Tofu Scramble:

2 cups cooked black beans

16 ounces tofu, firm, pressed, drained

1 chopped red pepper

1 1/2 cups sliced button mushrooms

1/2 of white onion, chopped

1 teaspoon minced garlic

1 tablespoon olive oil

Directions:

Take a skillet pan, place it over medium-high heat, add oil and when hot, add onion, pepper, mushrooms, and garlic and cook for 8 minutes until golden. Meanwhile, prepare the spice mix and for this, place all its ingredients in a bowl and stir until combined. When vegetables have cooked, add tofu in it, crumble it, then add black beans, sprinkle with prepared spice mix, stir and cook for 8 minutes until hot. Serve straight away

Chickpeas On Toast

Preparation time: 5 minutes

Cooking time: 15 minutes

Servings: 6

Ingredients:

14-oz cooked chickpeas

1 cup baby spinach

1/2 cup chopped white onion

1 cup crushed tomatoes

½ teaspoon minced garlic

¼ teaspoon ground black pepper

1/2 teaspoon brown sugar

1 teaspoon smoked paprika powder

1/3 teaspoon sea salt

1 tablespoon olive oil

6 slices of gluten-free bread, toasted

Directions:

Take a frying pan, place it over medium heat, add oil and when hot, add onion and cook for 2 minutes. Then stir in garlic, cook for 30 seconds until fragrant, stir in paprika and continue cooking for 10 seconds. Add tomatoes, stir, bring the mixture to simmer, season with black pepper, sugar, and salt and then stir in chickpeas. Sir, in spinach, cook for 2 minutes until leaves have wilted, then remove the pan from heat and taste to adjust seasoning. Serve cooked chickpeas on toasted bread

Chickpea Omelet

Preparation time: 5 minutes

Cooking time: 10 minutes

Servings: 1

Ingredients:

3 Tablespoon chickpea flour

1 small white onion, peeled, diced

½ teaspoon black salt

2 tablespoons chopped the dill

2 tablespoons chopped basil

1/8 teaspoon ground black pepper

2 Tablespoon olive oil

8 Tablespoon water

Directions:

Take a bowl, add flour in it along with salt and black pepper, stir until mixed, and then whisk in water until creamy. Take a skillet pan, place it over medium heat, add 1 tablespoon oil and when hot, add onion and cook for 4 minutes until cooked. Add onion to omelet mixture and then stir until combined. Add remaining oil into the pan, pour in prepared batter, spread evenly, and cook for 3 minutes per side until cooked. Serve omelet with bread.

Apple Pancakes

Preparation time: 15 minutes

Cooking time: 4 minutes

Servings: 4

Ingredients:

1 cup whole-wheat flour

¾ tsp. ground cinnamon, divided

¼ tsp. baking soda

1 tsp. baking powder

Pinch salt

1 egg

¾ cup ricotta cheese

1 cup buttermilk

1 tsp. vanilla extract

1 tbsp. sugar and 1 tsp. sugar, divided

1 apple, sliced into rings

4 tsp. butter

4 tsp. walnut oil

Directions:

In a bowl, mix the flour, ½ teaspoon cinnamon, baking soda, baking powder and salt. In another bowl, beat the eggs and stir in the cheese, milk, vanilla and 1 tablespoon sugar. Gradually add the second bowl to the first one. Mix well. Combine the remaining cinnamon and 1 teaspoon sugar in a separate dish. Coat each apple ring with this mixture. Pour the butter and oil in a pan over medium heat. Add the apples and pour the batter around the apple. Cook for 2 minutes. Flip and cook for another 2 minutes.

Quinoa Sensation Early Morning Porridge

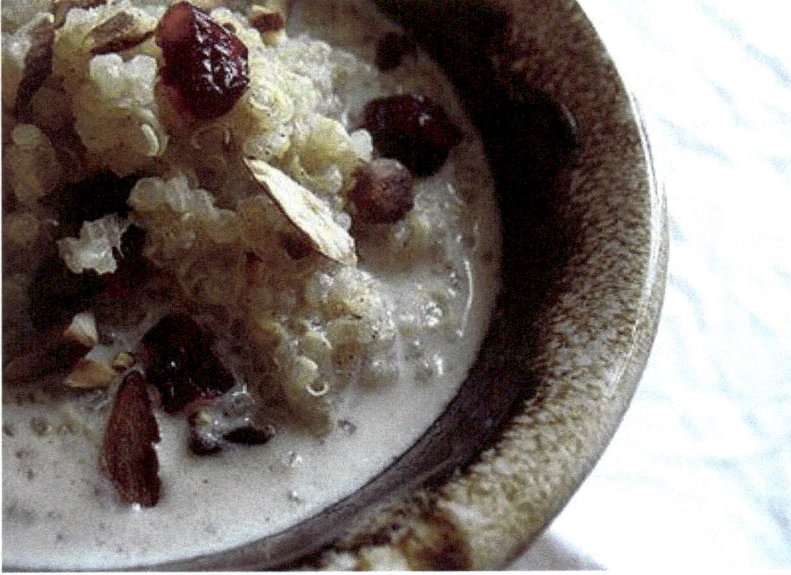

Preparation time: 5 minutes

Cooking time: 10 minutes

Servings: 3

Ingredients:

½ cup quinoa

3 tbsp. brown sugar

½ tsp. cinnamon

2 cups almond milk

½ cup water dash of salt

Directions:

Begin by heating the quinoa in a saucepan over medium heat. Add the cinnamon, and cook the quinoa until it's sufficiently toasted. This should take about five minutes. Afterwards, add the remaining ingredients. Bring the mixture to a boil. Next, place the stovetop to low heat, and allow the mixture to simmer for thirty minutes. If you need to, you can add more water if the porridge dries too quickly. Make sure to stir every few seconds. Enjoy!

Pita Bread

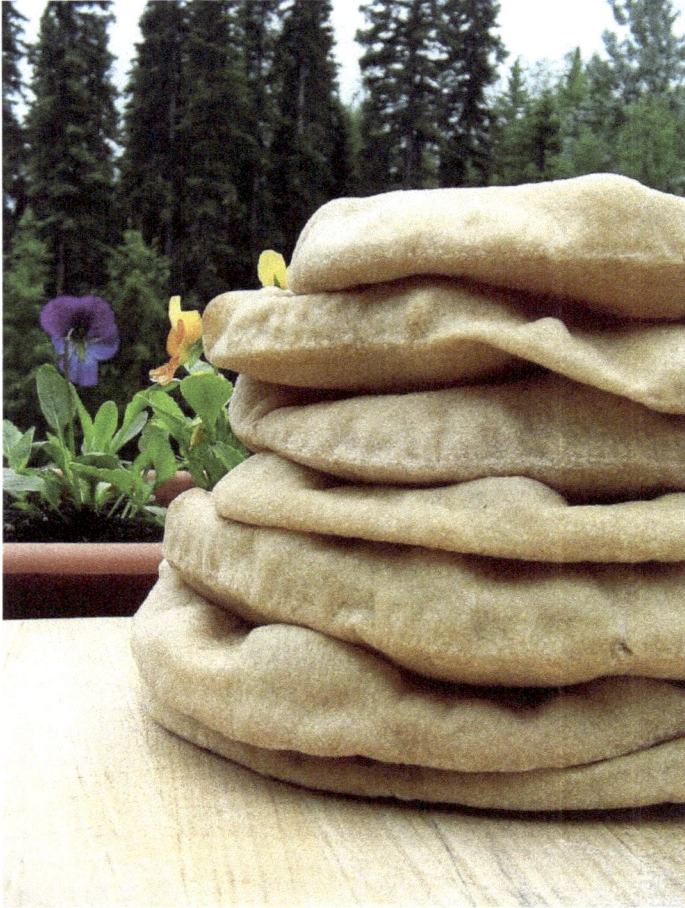

Servings: 8 pitas

Preparation time: 15 mins

Cooking time: 6 mins

Ingredients:

2 cups whole wheat flour

1 cup all-purpose flour

2½ teaspoons quick-acting yeast

1½ cups + 2 tablespoons lukewarm water

1 tablespoon olive oil

Directions:

Add all the dry Ingredients into a large bowl. Keep the east as far as possible from the salt. Add in the olive oil and enough of the water to make a firm, smooth dough. You might not need all of the water or you might need more, it depends on the humidity levels and brand of flour. Stir well until the all the flour is absorbed, to form a shaggy dough. Scrape the dough onto a clean, dry surface. Oil the work surface and hands with some olive oil. This will make the dough easier to handle while kneading. Knead for 7 - 10 minutes, until the dough becomes smoother and less sticky. Keep going until the dough slowly but easily bounces back to shape when poked. Divide the dough into 8 portions. Roll each piece about 3mm thick. Place on a lightly floured baking sheet and cover with clean, dry-damp kitchen towels. Rest for 30 minutes. Preheat the oven to 500 degrees Fahrenheit and after 30 minutes uncover the pitas and gently flip over. You will need to peel the breads off the baking tray but they'll come up easily as the tray is floured. Bake for 5 - 6 minutes until they are puffed but not at all colored. Cover with a kitchen towel and leave to coo. These pita breads will soften as they cool. Recipe Notes: These Pita Breads keep well for 2 - 3 days but can also be frozen. Place in a Ziploc bag and seal. To reheat pop straight in the oven from frozen at 350 degrees Fahrenheit for about 5 minutes. The salt in this recipe is optional. Omitting it will affect the flavor slightly, but not the recipe. The oil is also optional. If you omit it, add an extra tablespoon of water to compensate. If you do not add oil to the recipe the pita bread won't be as soft and will stale slightly quicker as oil is a preservative. Without oil, its best to freeze the breads and then reheat them when you need them.

Carrotastic Apple Muffins

Preparation time: 5 minutes

Cooking time: 40 minutes

Servings: 12.

Ingredients:
2 ¾ cups all-purpose flour
4 tsp. baking soda
1 cup brown sugar
1/3 cup white sugar
4 tsp. cinnamon
2 tsp. salt
1 tsp. baking powder
2 ½ cups grated carrots
2 cored, peeled, and shredded apples
1 1/3 cups applesauce
1/3 cup vegetable oil
6 tsp. dry egg replacer

Directions:

Begin by preheating your oven to 375 degrees Fahrenheit. Next, mix together the two sugars, the baking soda, the baking powder, the flour, the cinnamon, and the salt. Stir well. To the side, mix together the applesauce, the egg substitute, and the oil. Stir well, and add the dry ingredients to the wet ingredients. Spoon this created mixture into muffin tins, and bake the muffins for twenty minutes. Allow them to cool prior to serving, and enjoy!

Apple Oatmeal

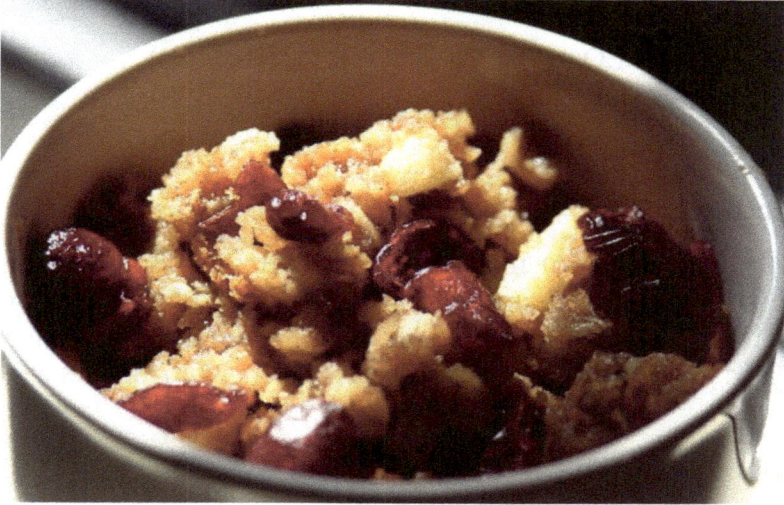

Preparation time: 5 minutes

Cooking time: 20 minutes

Servings: 4

Ingredients:

¼ Teaspoon Sea Salt

1 Cup Cashew Milk

1 Cup Strawberries, Halved & Fresh

1 Tablespoon Brown Sugar

2 Cups Apples, Diced

3 Cups Water

¼ Teaspoon Coconut Oil

½ Cup Steel Cut Oats

Directions:

Start by greasing your instant pot with oil, and add everything to it except for the milk and berries. Lock the lid and cook on high pressure for ten minutes. Allow for a natural pressure release, and then add in your milk and strawberries. Mix well, and serve warm

Creamy Roasted Plums

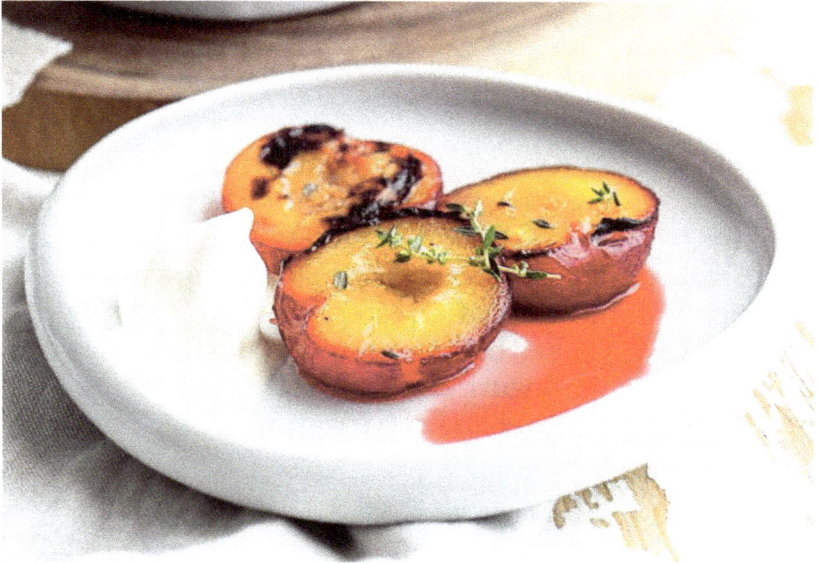

Preparation time: 5 minutes

Cooking time: 30 minutes

Servings: 3

Ingredients:

1 teaspoon olive oil

4 ripe plums, halved and pitted

4 teaspoons sugar

1 cup vanilla yogurt

2 tablespoons fresh basil, finely chopped

1 teaspoon honey

Directions:

Preheat the oven to 400°F. Oil a large baking dish. Place the plums inside, cut side up, and sprinkle ½ teaspoon sugar over each. Bake, uncovered, for 35 minutes. While the plums are baking, stir together the yogurt, basil, and honey. Divide half of yogurt mixture onto each of 4 plates, or a large serving platter. When plums are finished baking, remove them from the oven and place 2 halves over yogurt on each plate. Fill the holes with remaining yogurt mixture and serve warm.

Italian Frittata

Preparation time: 5 minutes

Cooking time: 40 minutes

Servings: 3

Ingredients:

6 large eggs, beaten

¼ cup extra-virgin olive oil

1 cup shitake mushrooms, cut very thin

½ medium yellow onion, cut very thin slices

1 large leeks, white and light green parts rinsed, chopped finely

8 basil leaves, torn

¼ cup Pecorino Romano, grated

1 teaspoon Unrefined Sea salt

Directions:

Preheat the oven to 350°F. Heat the oil in a large, wide, ovenproof skillet over medium-high heat. Add the onion and sauté, stirring occasionally, until softened and golden, 4 minutes. Add mushrooms and brown them, 4 minutes. Add the leeks, stir, and cook for another 4 minutes. Add the basil leaves, beaten eggs, Pecorino Romano, and salt. Mix well and reduce heat to medium-low. Cook, undisturbed, for 4 to 5 minutes, or until the eggs are cooked through. Finish off the frittata by putting the skillet in the oven until the frittata top is golden and the eggs are set. Cut into 4 and serve.

Mango Chia Smoothie

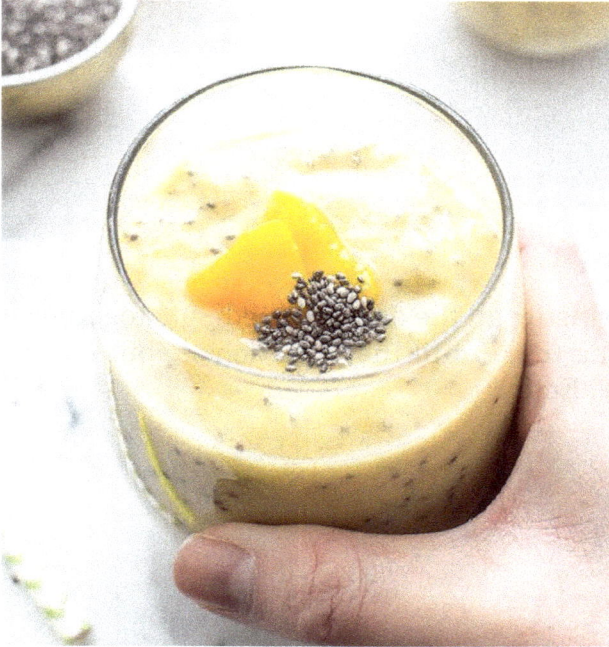

Preparation time: 5 minutes

Cooking time: 0 minutes

1 Smoothie.

Ingredients:
1 peeled and chopped mango
1 sliced banana

1 tsp. flax seeds

½ tbsp. chia seeds

1 cup water

½ cup romaine lettuce

3 ice cubes

Directions:

Begin by bringing all the above ingredients together in a blender and blending them until they've reached your desired smoothie consistency. Enjoy!

Breakfast Protein Bars

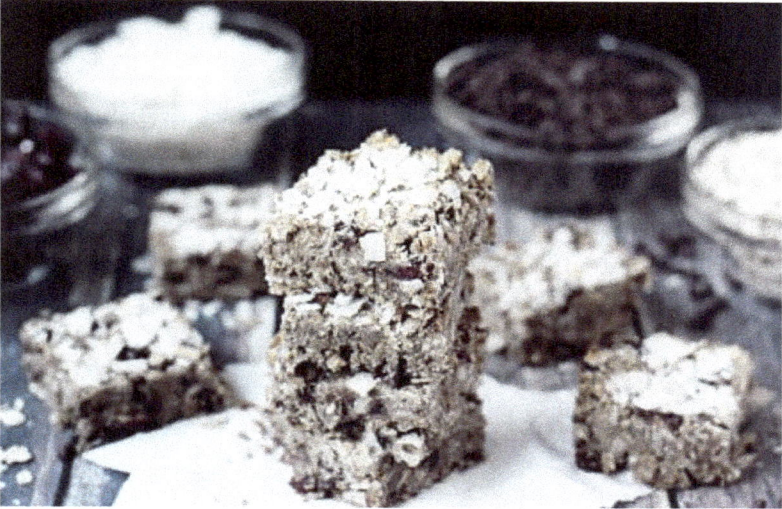

Servings: 16

Preparation time: 35 min

INGREDIENTS:

1 cup cashew cheese spread

2 tbsp. softened cocoa butter

4 tbsp. coconut flour

½ cup full fat coconut milk

2 scoops vegan protein powder

¼ teaspoon stevia

1 tsp. vanilla extract

Total number of Ingredients: 7

Directions:

Preheat oven to 375°F. Whisk together cocoa butter, cashew cheese spread, stevia, and coconut milk until mixed well. Stir the coconut flour and protein powder through until completely combined. Pour into a baking sheet lined with parchment paper, and bake for 30 minutes until the batter has set. Let it cool, and slice into 16 bars. Can be stored chilled for a week or frozen up to 2 months.

Poached Eggs

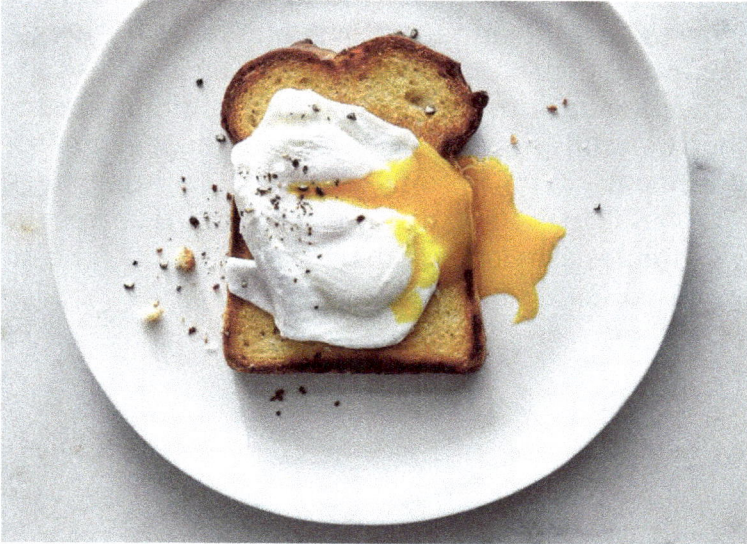

Preparation time: 5 minutes

Cooking time: 30 minutes

Servings: 3

Ingredients:

1 large egg

1 teaspoon kosher salt

2 teaspoons of white vinegar

Directions:

Place water in a deep 2-quart saucier until the water level is at an inch up the sides. Add salt and white vinegar. Set heat to medium and bring water to a simmer. Crack one large fresh egg into a custard cup and then use a spoon or a spatula handle to stir water in one direction until you see i's smoothly spinning around like a whirlpool. Carefully drop the egg right into the center of the swirl. The movement of the water will keep the egg whites from spreading out. Turn off heat. Cover pan and then set timer for exactly 5 minutes. Do not disturb the pan in any way. Remove egg using a slotted spoon. Immediately serve.

Avocado Mug Bread

Preparation time: 2 min

Cooking time: 2 min

Servings: 1

Ingredients:
¼ cup Almond Flour

½ tsp Baking Powder

¼ tsp Salt

¼ cup Mashed Avocados

1 tbsp Coconut Oil

Directions:
Mix all Ingredients in a microwave-safe mug. Microwave for 90 seconds. Cool for 2 minutes.

Meat-Free Breakfast Chili

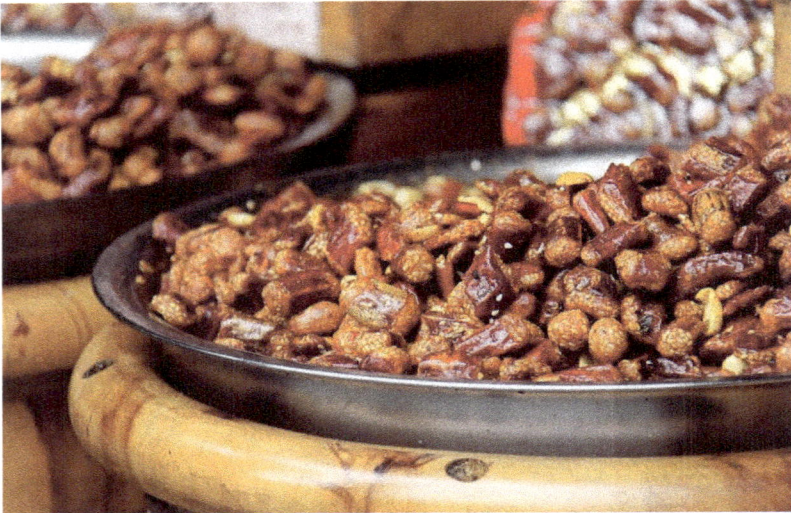

Preparation time: 10 minutes

Cooking time: 20 min

Servings: 4

Ingredients:

400 grams Textured-Vegetable Protein

¼ cup Red Kidney Beans

½ cup Canned Diced Tomatoes

1 Large Bell Pepper, diced

1 Large White Onion, diced

1 tsp Cumin Powder

1 tsp Chili Powder

1 tsp Paprika

1 tsp Garlic Powder

½ tsp Dried Oregano

2 cups Water

Directions:

Combine all Ingredients in a pot. Simmer for 20 minutes. Serve with your favorite bread or some slices of fresh avocado.

Apple Pancakes

Preparation time: 10 minutes

Cooking time: 16 minutes

Servings: 4

Ingredients:

1 and ¾ cups buckwheat flour

2 tablespoons coconut sugar

2 teaspoons baking powder

¼ teaspoon vanilla extract

2 teaspoons cinnamon powder

1 and ¼ cups almond milk

1 tablespoon flaxseed, ground mixed with 3 tablespoons water

1 cup apple, peeled, cored and chopped

A drizzle of vegetable oil

Directions:

In a bowl, mix flour with sugar, baking powder, vanilla extract and cinnamon and stir. Add flaxseed mix, milk and apple and stir well until you obtain your pancake batter. Grease your air fryer with the oil, spread ¼ of the batter, cover and cook at 360 degrees F for 5 minutes, flipping it halfway. Transfer pancake to a plate, repeat the process with the rest of the batter and serve them for breakfast. Enjoy!

Vegan Cheese Sandwich

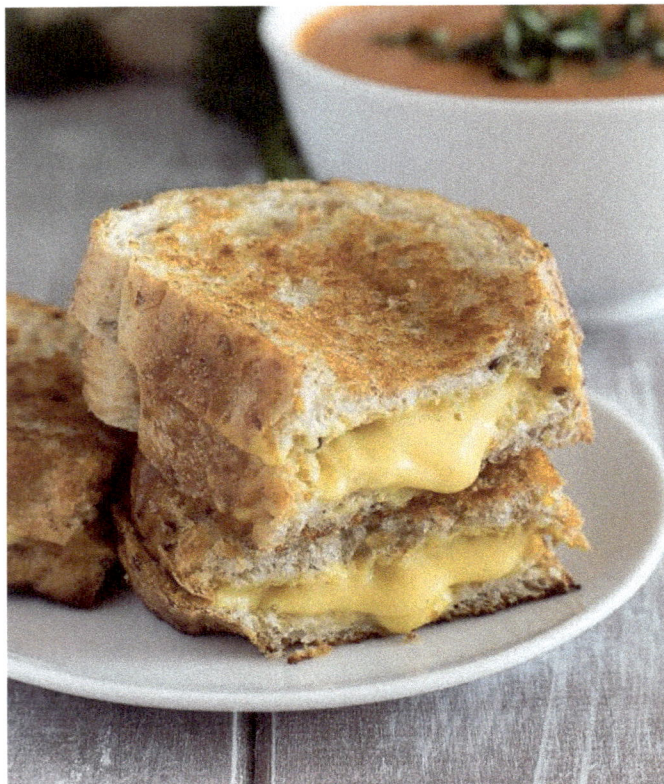

Preparation time: 10 minutes

Cooking time: 8 minutes

Servings: 1

Ingredients:

2 slices vegan bread

2 slices cashew cheese

2 teaspoons cashew butter

Directions:

Spread cashew butter on bread slices, add vegan cheese on one slice, top with the other, cut into halves diagonally, put in your air fryer, cover and cook at 370 degrees F for 8 minutes, flipping the sandwiches halfway. Serve them right away. Enjoy!

Onion and Tofu Mix

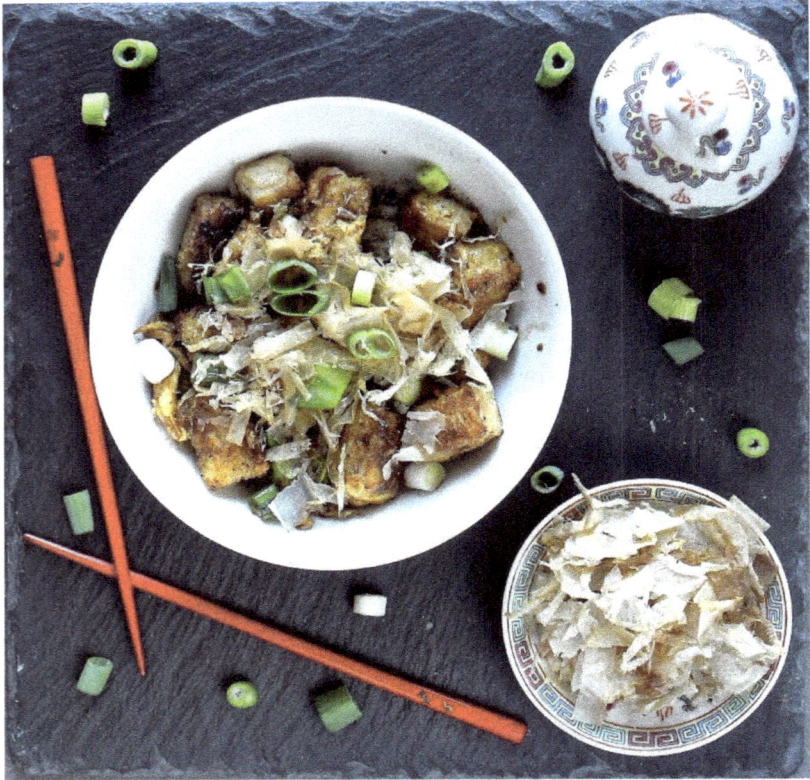

Preparation time: 10 minutes

Cooking time: 15 minutes

Servings: 2

Ingredients:

2 tablespoons flax meal mixed with 3 tablespoons water

1 yellow onion, sliced

1 teaspoon coconut aminos

Cooking spray

A pinch of black pepper

¼ cup firm tofu, cubed

Directions:

In a bowl, mix flax meal with coconut aminos and black pepper and whisk well. Grease your air fryer with the cooking spray, preheat at 350 degrees F, add onion slices and cook for 10 minutes. Add flax meal and tofu, cook for 5 minutes more, divide between 2 plates and serve for breakfast. Enjoy!

Vegan Sausage Patties

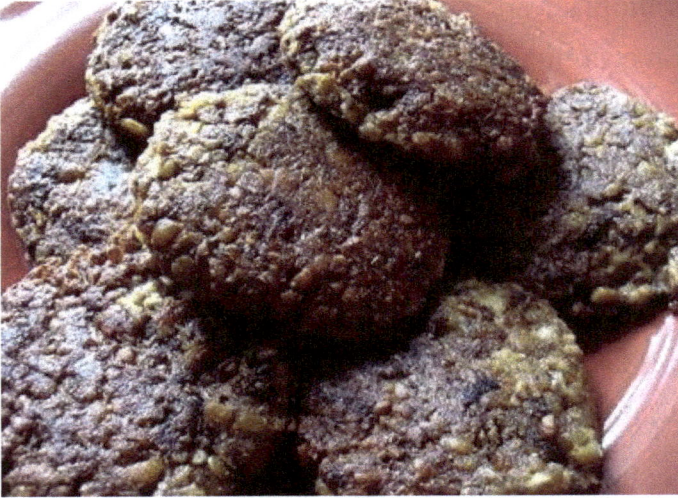

Preparation time: 10 minutes

Cooking time: 6 minutes

Servings: 4

Ingredients

1 1/2 tablespoon sausage spice blend

1 cup pecans or walnuts, chopped

1 cup chickpeas, drained and rinsed

Directions:

In a food processor, blend chickpeas and nuts until you have a chunky sort of paste. Plop the mixture into a bowl and stir in the spices until well incorporated. Cover the mixture and allow to set in the fridge for at least 30 minutes for flavors to blend together. In a pan placed on a stove, heat coconut or olive oil on medium-low heat. Make patties and cook them for around 10 minutes. Gently flip and cook the other side for another 10 minutes. Flip one more time and cook for 5 more minutes. Then remove from the pan and serve. You could also store them in freezer bags and freeze them to enjoy the sausages throughout the week.

Matcha Avocado Pancakes

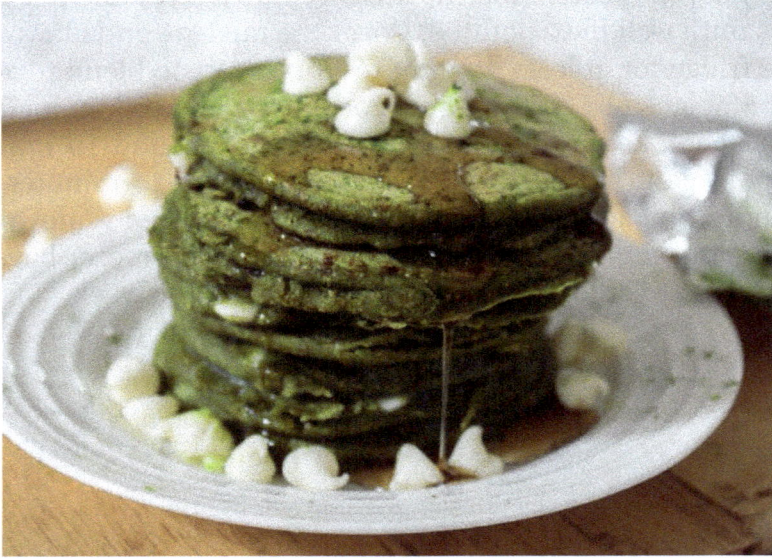

Preparation time: 10 minutes

Cooking time: 5 min

Servings: 6

Ingredients:

1 cup Almond Flour

1 medium-sized Avocado, mashed

1 cup Coconut Milk

1 tbsp Matcha Powder

½ tsp Baking Soda

¼ tsp Salt

Directions:

Mix all Ingredients into a batter. Add water, a tablespoon at a time, to thin out the mixture if needed. Lightly oil a nonstick pan. Ladle approximately 1/3 cup of the batter and cook over medium heat until bubbly on the surface (about 2-3 minutes). Flip the pancake over and cook for another minute.

Veggie Casserole

Preparation time: 10 minutes

Cooking time: 15 minutes

Servings: 2

Ingredients:
1 yellow onion, chopped
1 teaspoon garlic, minced
1 teaspoon olive oil
1 carrot, chopped
2 celery stalks, chopped
½ cup shiitake mushrooms, chopped
½ cup red bell pepper, chopped
Salt and black pepper to the taste
1 teaspoon oregano, dried
½ teaspoon red pepper flakes
½ teaspoon cumin, ground
½ teaspoon dill, dried
7 ounces firm tofu, cubed
1 tablespoon lemon juice
2 tablespoons water
½ cup quinoa, already cooked

2 tablespoons nutritional yeast

Directions:

Heat up a pan with the oil over medium-high heat, add garlic and onion, stir and cook for 3 minutes. Add bell pepper, celery and carrot, stir and cook for 3 minutes. Add salt, pepper, mushrooms, oregano, dill, cumin and pepper flakes, stir and cook for 3 minutes more. In your food processor, mix tofu with yeast, lemon juice and water and blend well. Add quinoa and blend again. Add sautéed veggies, stir gently pour everything into your air fryer's pan and cook everything at 350 degrees F for 15 minutes. Divide your breakfast casserole between plates and serve. Enjoy!

Navy Bean and Jalapeno Pepper Soup

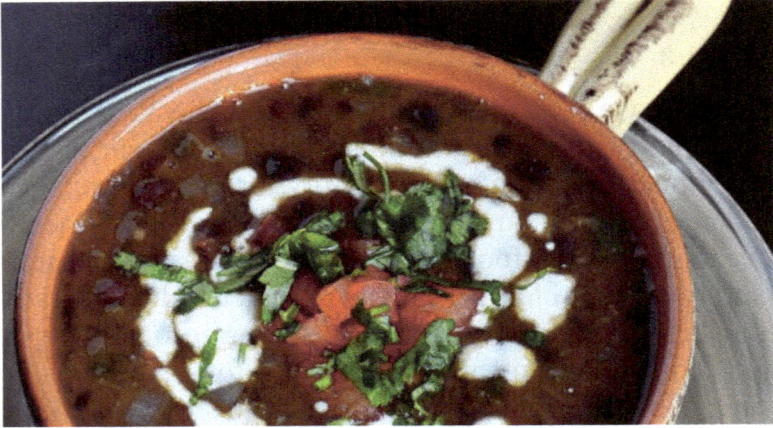

Ingredients:

1 teaspoon olive oil

1/2 cup chopped red onions

4 cloves garlic, minced

1 cup vegetable broth

1 cup vegetable stock

1 cup salsa

1 14-ounce can navy beans

1 green bell pepper, chopped

1 jalapeno pepper, coarsely chopped

1/2 teaspoon sea salt

1 avocado, chopped

1/2 cup loosely-packed cilantro

Directions:

Optional: 1/2 cup crumbled corn tortilla chips Add olive oil to a pan and heat it to medium. Add red onions and garlic to saucepan and sauté until softened. Add the stock, salsa, bell peppers, jalapeno, beans, and sea salt. Bring to a boil over high heat. Reduce to low and simmer for 5 minutes. Garnish with half of the avocado, cilantro, and tortilla chips.

Oriental Garlic and Parsnip Soup

Ingredients

1 tablespoon sesame seed oil

2 teaspoon crushed garlic

1 tablespoon chopped fresh cilantro

1 teaspoon chili garlic sauce

3 red onions, chopped

3 large parsnips, peeled and sliced

Sea salt to taste

5 cups vegetable broth

Directions:

Heat oil over medium heat. Cook the garlic, cilantro and chili garlic sauce. Stir fry the onion until tender. Add the parsnips and potato. Cook for 5 minutes and add the vegetable broth. Simmer until potatoes and parsnips are soft. Blend until smooth.

Italian Squash and Potato Soup

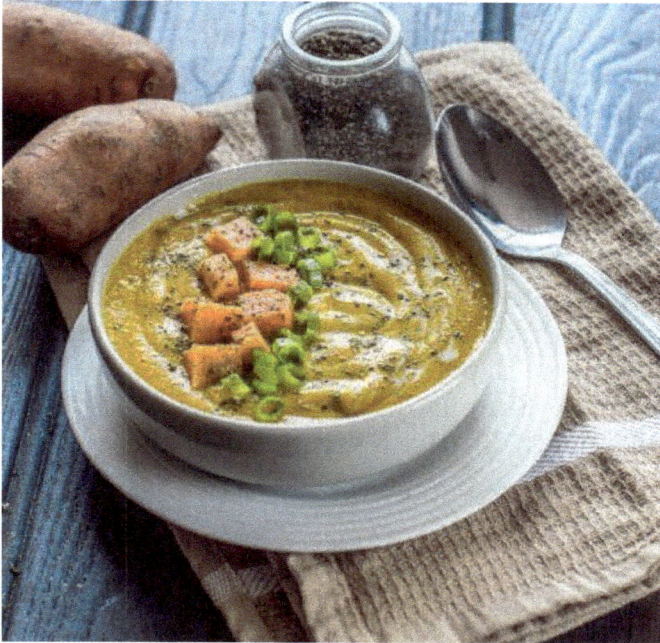

Ingredients

1 tablespoon extra virgin olive oil

2 teaspoon crushed garlic

½ tsp. dried basil

1 teaspoon Italian seasoning

1 red onion, chopped

3 large winter squash, peeled and sliced

Sea salt to taste

1 large potato, peeled and chopped

5 cups vegetable broth

Directions:

Heat oil over medium heat. Cook the garlic, dried basil and Italian seasoning. Stir fry the onion until tender. Add the winter squash and potato. Cook for 5 minutes and add the vegetable broth. Simmer until potatoes and winter squash are soft. Blend until smooth. Turnip and Parsnip Soup Ingredients 1 tablespoon non-dairy butter 2 teaspoon crushed garlic 1 teaspoon dried thyme 1 red onion, chopped 1 large turnip, peeled and sliced 1 large parsnip, peeled and sliced Sea salt to taste 1 large potato, peeled and chopped 5 cups vegetable broth Vegan cheese slices, for topping Heat and melt non-dairy butter over medium heat. Cook the garlic, and thyme. Stir fry the onion until tender. Add the turnip, parsnip and potato. Cook for 5 minutes and add the vegetable broth. Simmer until potatoes and turnips are soft. Blend until smooth. Top with vegan cheese slices

Smoky Summer Squash and Onion Soup

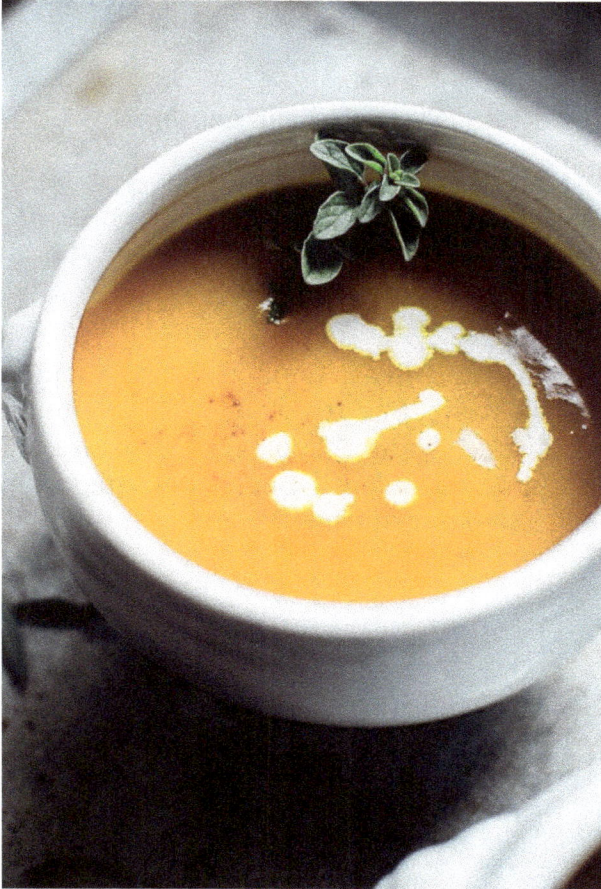

Ingredients

1 tablespoon extra virgin olive oil

2 teaspoon crushed garlic

1 tablespoon chopped fresh cilantro

1 teaspoon ground annatto

½ tsp. cumin

3 red onions, chopped

3 pcs. small summer squash, peeled and sliced

Sea salt to taste

1 large butternut squash, peeled and chopped

5 cups vegetable broth

Directions:

Heat oil over medium heat. Cook the garlic, annatto, cumin, cilantro and chili paste. Stir fry the onion until tender. Add the summer squash and potato. Cook for 5 minutes and add the vegetable broth. Simmer until butternut squash and summer squash are soft. Blend until smooth.

Buttery Poblano Pepper Soup

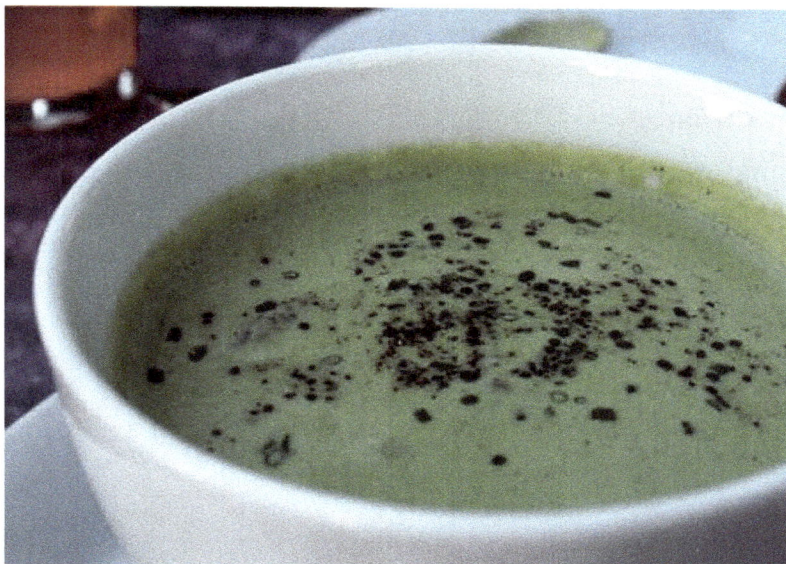

Ingredients

4 tablespoons organic butter

1 small red onion, coarsely chopped

1 large leek, white part only, sliced

1 green bell pepper, coarsely chopped

1 (or two if you like things spicy) small dry-roasted poblano chili, sliced

4 cloves garlic, diced

1 large sweet potato, cubed (you can use two if you like your soup thick)

4 cups vegetable broth

1 cup almonds

1-1/4 cup almond milk

Sea Salt Black pepper, to taste

Directions:

Optional garnish: Sliced jalapeno pepper Soak the cashews in almond milk for half an hour. Melt non-dairy butter in a pan. Cook the onion, leek, chilies, red bell pepper, garlic, and potato over low heat until the onion is translucent. Add the broth into the pan. Simmer until the potatoes are fork tender, about 25 min. Remove from the heat. Pour into a blender and blend until smooth. Clean the blender. Blend cashews with the milk until smooth Stir this into the soup. Heat on medium for a few minutes. Garnish with slices of jalapeno chili.

Lebanese Inspired Winter Squash Soup

Ingredients

4 tablespoons salted butter

1 small red onion, coarsely chopped

1 large leek, white part only, sliced

1 green bell pepper, coarsely chopped

1 (or two if you like things spicy) small dry-roasted poblano chili, sliced

4 cloves garlic, diced

1 small winter squash, cubed (you can use two if you like your soup thick)

4 cups vegetable broth

2 tsp. cumin

2 tsp. cinnamon

Juice of 1 lemon

1 cup almonds

1-1/4 cup almond milk

Sea Salt Black pepper, to taste

Directions:

Optional garnish: Sliced jalapeno pepper Soak the cashews in almond milk for half an hour. Melt non-dairy butter in a pan. Cook the onion, leek, chilies, red bell pepper, garlic, and squash over low heat until the onion is translucent. Add the broth, cumin, cinnamon and lemon juice into the pan. Simmer until the squash are fork tender, about 25 min. Remove from the heat. Pour into a blender and blend until smooth. Clean the blender. Blend cashews with the milk until smooth Stir this into the soup. Heat on medium for a few minutes. Garnish with slices of jalapeno chili.

Fusion Red Potato Soup

Ingredients

4 tbsp. canola oil

4 tablespoons coconut cream

1 small red onion, coarsely chopped

1 large leek, white part only, sliced

1 green red pepper, coarsely chopped

1 (or two if you like things spicy) small dry-roasted poblano chili, sliced

9 cloves garlic, diced

1 large red potato, cubed (you can use two if you like your soup thick)

4 cups vegetable broth

3 pcs. Thai basil, coarsely chopped

2 tsp. Sriracha hot sauce

5 Thai bird chilies

1 tsp. curry powder

1 cup almonds

1-1/4 cup coconut milk

Sea Salt Black pepper, to taste

Directions:

Optional garnish: Sliced Thai bird chilies Soak the cashews in almond milk for half an hour. Heat oil in a pan. Cook the onion, leek, chilies, red bell pepper, garlic, and potato over low heat until the onion is translucent. Add the broth, basil, Sriracha hot sauce, curry powder & Thai bird chilies into the pan. Simmer until the potatoes are fork tender, about 25 min. Remove from the heat. Pour into a blender and blend until smooth. Clean the blender. Blend cashews with the coconut cream and milk until smooth Stir this into the soup. Heat on medium for a few minutes. Garnish with slices of Thai bird chilies.

Creamy Potato and Leek Soup

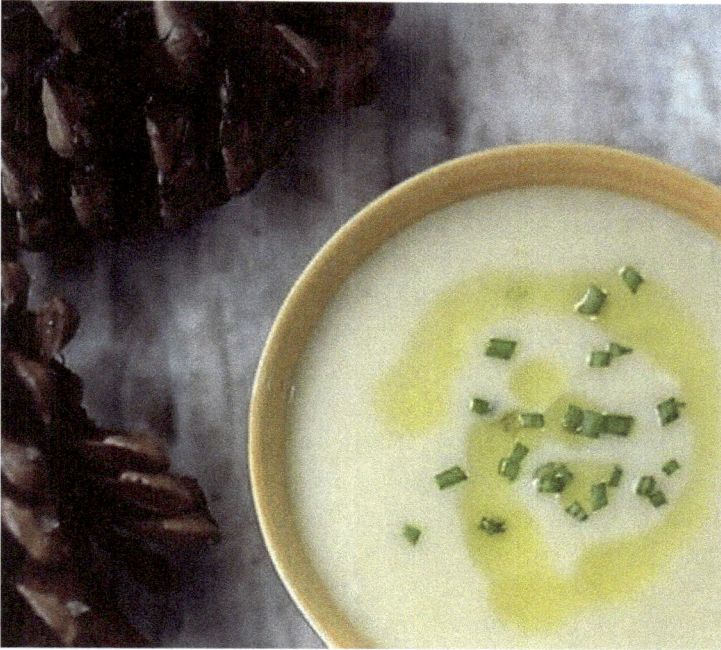

Ingredients:

4 tablespoons salted butter

1 small red onion, coarsely chopped

1 large leek, white part only, sliced

1 (or two if you like things spicy) small dry-roasted poblano chili, sliced

8 cloves garlic, diced

1 large potato, cubed (you can use two if you like your soup thick)

4 cups vegetable broth

1 cup cashews

1-1/4 cup almond milk

Sea Salt Black pepper, to taste

Directions:

Optional garnish: Sliced jalapeno pepper Soak the cashews in almond milk for half an hour. Melt non-dairy butter in a pan. Cook the onion, leek, chilies, red bell pepper, garlic, and potato over low heat until the onion is translucent. Add the broth into the pan. Simmer until the potatoes are fork tender, about 25 min. Remove from the heat. Pour into a blender and blend until smooth. Clean the blender. Blend cashews with the milk until smooth Stir this into the soup. Heat on medium for a few minutes. Garnish with slices of jalapeno chili.

www.ingramcontent.com/pod-product-compliance
Lightning Source LLC
Chambersburg PA
CBHW070734030426
42336CB00013B/1967